THE SENSES

BODYWORKS

Tracy Maurer

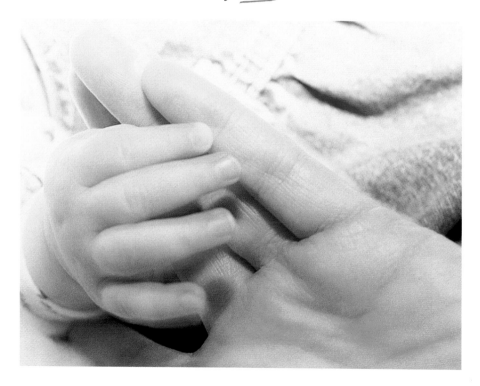

The Rourke Corporation, Inc.
Vero Beach, Florida 32964

Tracy M. Maurer specializes in non-fiction and business writing. Her most recently published children's books include the Let's Dance Series, also from Rourke Publishing.

With appreciation to Lois M. Nelson, Paige Henson, Drew and Tracy McCroen, and John and Jennifer Atwater.

PHOTO CREDITS:
© Lois M. Nelson: title page, page 12; © Timothy L. Vacula: cover, pages 4, 8, 13, 15, 17, 21; © Diane Farleo: page 18

ILLUSTRATIONS: © Todd Tennyson: pages 7, 10

EDITORIAL SERVICES: Janice L. Smith for Penworthy Learning Systems

612.8
MAU

1- 02

1304760

Library of Congress Cataloging-in-Publication Data

Maurer, Tracy, 1965-
    The senses / by Tracy Maurer.
        p. cm. — (Bodyworks)
    Summary: Describes the five senses and how they work through various parts of the body to tell us about the world outside ourselves.
    ISBN 0-86593-583-1
    1. Senses and sensation Juvenile literature. [1. Senses and sensation.]
I. Title. II. Series: Maurer, Tracy, 1965- Bodyworks.
QP434.M38 1999
612.8—dc21   99-23382
                                                                    CIP

Printed in the USA

TABLE OF CONTENTS

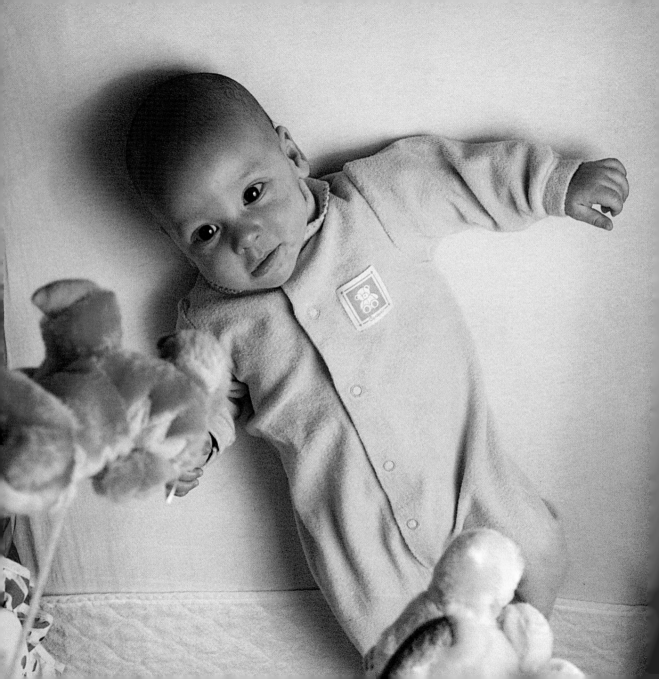

YOU ARE HERE

Touch, sight, sound, smell, and taste tell you about the world outside your body. These **senses** (SENS ez) also tell you about your body's position. Are you sitting on a chair or standing on your head? Check your five senses.

Your senses send billions of signals to your brain every few seconds. Your brain deals with just a few signals at a time. If it took in all the signals at once, you would go crazy!

Babies learn about the world through their senses.

THE CONTROL CENTER

Your brain is the control center for your senses. Signals travel to your brain along thin cords called **nerves** (NERVZ). These signals can zoom along at up to 290 miles (470 kilometers) per hour.

Your brain gives meanings to signals that come in. It also sends signals out to the body. If you step on a pin, your brain knows the signals from your foot mean pain. It zaps a signal back to your foot telling it to pull away quickly. This is a **reflex** (REE FLEKS) action. Your body moves on its own.

Each of the five senses sends signals to a certain part of the brain.

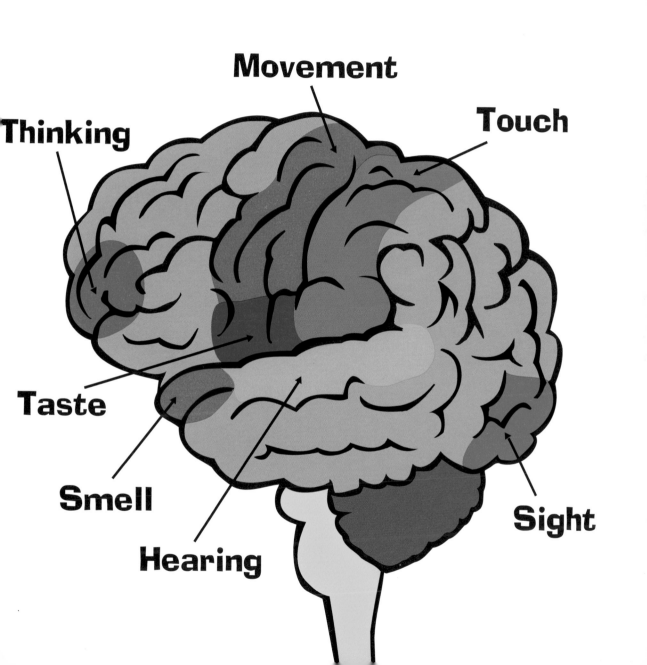

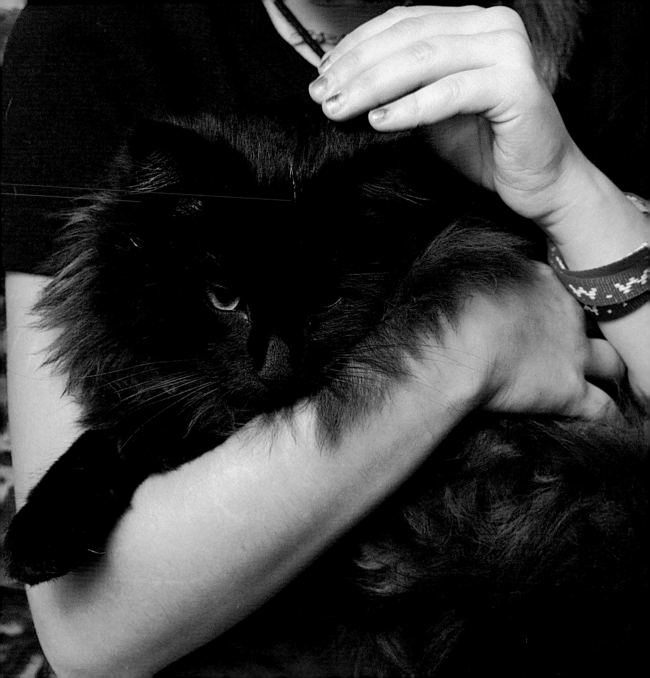

TOUCH

Touch tells you how things feel. Is a cat's fur soft or rough? Is this book heavy or light? Is your nose warm or cold?

Humans need to touch each other. Babies grow better when they're held often. Adults shake hands to greet each other. Some even hug and kiss.

You mainly use skin to touch things. Some places on the body sense touch better than others. Your fingertips sense touch very well. So do the soles of your feet. That's why your feet are so ticklish.

What you touch can change how you feel. Petting a cat can make you feel calm.

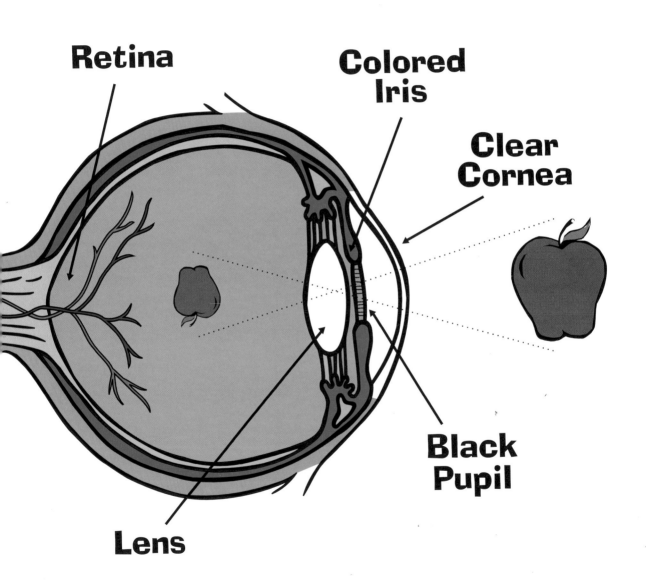

SIGHT

Everything you see is light. Light shines upside down on the **retina** (RET n uh) at the back of the eyeball. The retina changes the light into signals. These signals speed to the brain. The brain quickly reads them and forms right-side-up images.

Your eyes move very fast all the time. A group of six muscles lets them look in every direction. Both eyes move together, but each one sees things a bit differently. Your brain overlaps **images** (IM ij ez) from each eye to make one picture.

Images shine in upside down. The brain flips the images back up.

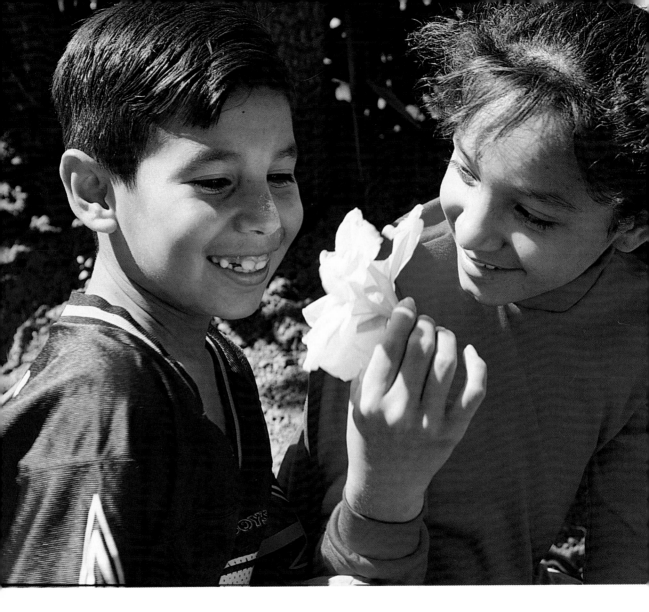

What senses do you think these children are using?

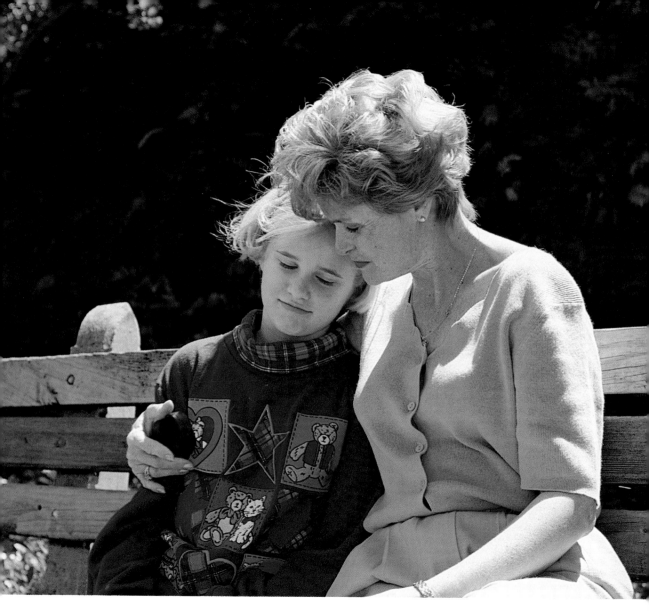

A hug can make you feel good. Humans need to touch each other.

SOUND

All sounds come from **sound waves** (SOWND WAYVZ). The number of waves combined with the size of the waves create each sound.

Your ears catch sound waves. The eardrum and three middle ear bones turn the waves into signals. The brain receives the signals and sorts them. You hear what is important to you. A friend calling your name or a favorite song may get your attention. Other sounds become noise.

Big sound waves are loud. Small ones are quiet. What size sound waves do you think a whisper makes?

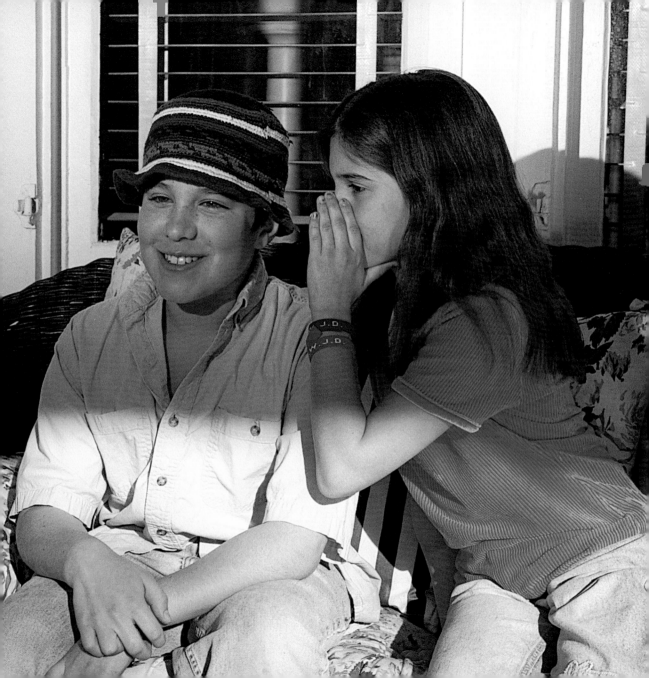

SMELL

You sense **odors** (O durz) best when you breathe in. Think of a grocery scanner "reading" prices. Your nose reads odors with the dime-sized **epithelium** (EP uh THEE lee um) in each **nostril** (NAHS tril). The epitheliums help change odors into signals to send to your brain.

You can smell much better than you can taste. You can also remember odors very well—some 10,000 of them. You don't need to see a skunk to know when one has sprayed!

You can remember some odors long after you smell them. Once you smell a rose, you can tell it from other flowers.

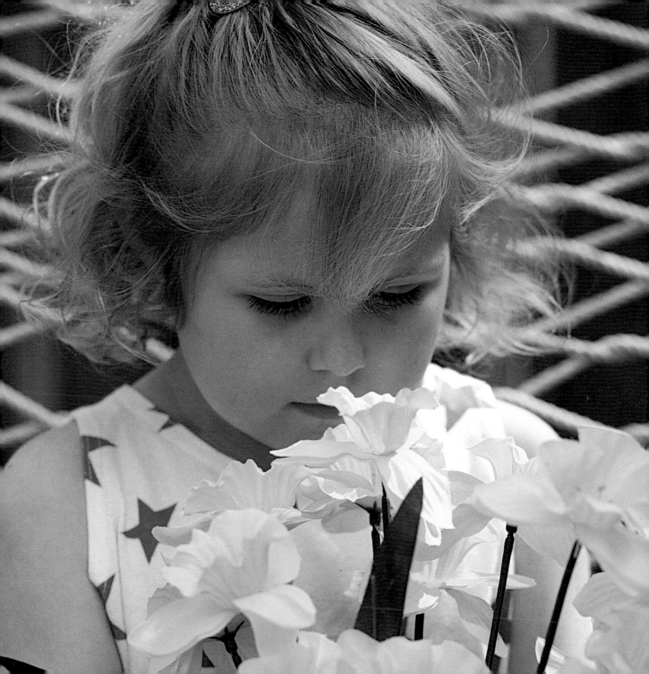

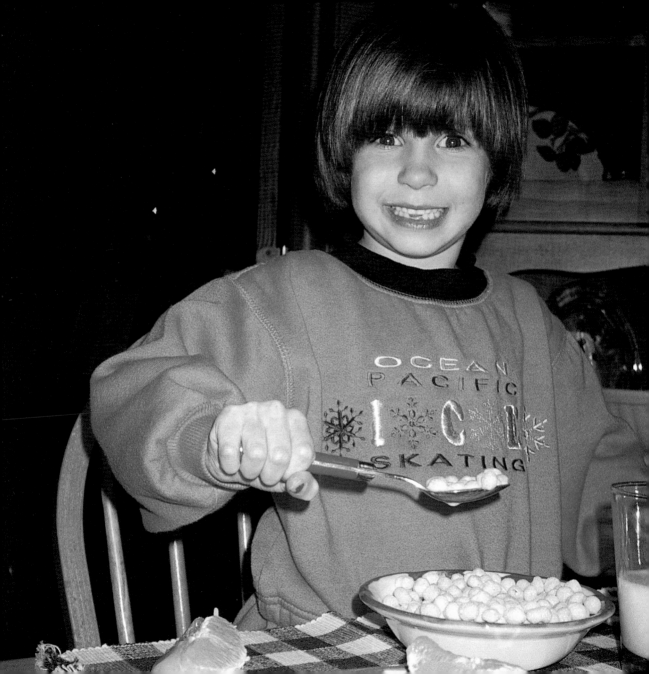

TASTE

The tongue knows only four basic tastes: sweet, salty, sour, and bitter. Different parts of the tongue respond to each taste. The tip senses sweet and salty. The sides sense sour and the back senses bitter. About 10,000 tiny **tastebuds** (TAYST BUDZ) dot the tongue's bumps.

Taste buds send signals to the brain. Your brain senses **flavor** (FLAY vur) based on many factors. These include how strong the tastes seem, how they smell, and how they feel. That's why you can taste the difference between a lemon and lemonade.

Children have more taste buds than adults, because taste buds die with age.

SENSING SAFETY

Signals from many senses help keep you safe. Before you cross the street, you look for cars. You also listen for motors. You might feel the wind from cars rushing by or smell diesel fuel from a truck.

When a person loses one sense, the other four senses take over. Blind people depend on touch to give them images. Deaf people carefully watch others' lips to "read" sounds.

Even while you play, your senses work to protect you. Sight keeps you from falling. Touch keeps you off hot metal.

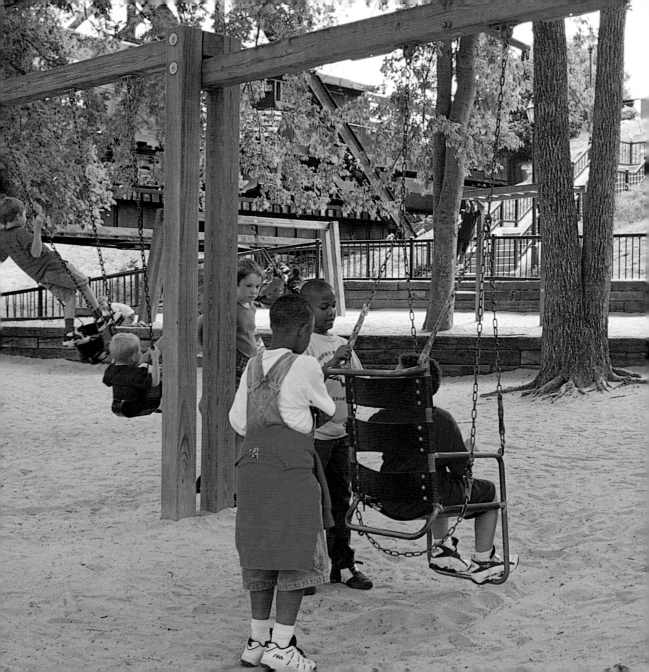

ENJOYING YOUR SENSES

Your senses protect you, as you should protect them. Wear sunglasses when you play in bright sunlight. Rest your eyes after spending time in front of a computer or television. Listen to music at a low volume. Loud sounds can hurt your eardrums forever.

Take time to enjoy your senses. Smell flowers. Taste new foods. Hug a friend. Watch ants. Hear birds chirping. Your senses bring you the world!

GLOSSARY

epithelium (EP uh THEE lee um) — in the nose, it is a layer of cells that helps change odors into signals to send to your brain

flavor (FLAY vur) — the mix of taste, smell, and texture

images (IM ij ez) — mental pictures

nerves (NERVZ) — thin fibers that send signals to and from the brain

nostril (NAHS tril) — opening of the nose

odors (O durz) — smells

reflex (REE FLEKS) — quick body movements that happen on their own

retina (RET n uh) — the inside wall at the back of the eyeball

senses (SENS ez) — sight, touch, hearing, taste, smell

sound waves (SOWND WAYVZ) — pulses on which sound travels

taste buds (TAYST BUDZ) — cells on the tongue's bumps that sense flavors

INDEX

FURTHER READING:

Find out more about Bodyworks with these helpful books:

• Walker, Richard. *The Children's Atlas of the Human Body.* Brookfield, Connecticut: The Millbrook Press, 1994.
• Miller, Jonathan, and David Pelham. *The Human Body: The Classic Three-Dimensional Book.* New York: Penguin Books, 1983.
• Williams, Dr. Frances. *Inside Guides: Human Body.* New York: DK Publishing, 1997.

On CD-ROM
• *The Family Doctor,* 3rd Edition. Edited by Allan H. Bruckheim, M.D. © Creative Multimedia, 1993-1994.